PCOS Palate

Nourishing Recipes for Wellness

Rose Gruet

Chapter One

Nourishing Recipes for Wellness

purpose of this book

The book's goal is to offer healthy recipes specifically designed for people with PCOS.

In order to give people with PCOS (polycystic ovarian syndrome) a comprehensive resource of nourishing recipes specifically designed to support their health and well-being, the book "PCOS Palate: Nourishing Recipes for Wellness" was written. In order to address the special dietary requirements and difficulties that people with PCOS encounter, the book provides enticing and nourishing recipes that support insulin sensitivity, hormone balance, weight control, and general metabolic health

A succinct description of PCOS

Polycystic Ovary Syndrome, or PCOS, is a hormonal condition that affects many women who are fertile. Cysts in the ovaries, high androgen levels (male hormones), and irregular menstrual periods are its defining features. There is a wide range of symptoms that can include infertility, weight gain, acne, irregular periods, and excessive hair growth. Insulin resistance and metabolic disorders like type 2 diabetes and obesity are also linked to PCOS. Although the precise etiology of PCOS remains unclear, genetics, insulin resistance, and hormone imbalance are thought to be contributing factors. Management usually entails dietary and activity modifications, as well as prescription drugs to treat particular symptoms and, if desired, increase fertility.

Diet is important for controlling the symptoms of PCOS

Because diet has a direct impact

on hormone levels, insulin sensitivity, and general metabolic health, it is essential for managing PCOS symptoms. This is why diet is crucial for PCOS management:

1. Insulin Resistance: Insulin resistance is a common condition among PCOS-affected women. It is characterized by ineffective insulin response from cells, which raises blood sugar levels. Insulin resistance can be decreased and insulin sensitivity increased with a blood sugar-stabilizing diet.

2. Weight management: Obesity and weight gain are frequently linked to PCOS, which can worsen symptoms and raise the risk of consequences like type 2 diabetes and cardiovascular disease. By helping people with PCOS reach and maintain a healthy weight, a balanced diet can lessen the severity of symptoms and the chance of developing related health issues.

3. Hormonal Balance: Insulin, testosterone, and estrogen levels all of which are frequently out of balance in women with PCOS can be influenced by diet. A few meals can help control hormone production and lessen symptoms including irregular menstrual periods, acne, and excessive hair growth.

4. Chronic low-grade inflammation is linked to PCOS and may exacerbate insulin resistance and other metabolic disorders. Eating a diet high in whole grains, fruits, vegetables, healthy fats, and other anti-inflammatory foods can help lower inflammation and enhance general health.

5. Fertility: Diet can significantly improve fertility for women with PCOS who are attempting to conceive. To enhance the chances of ovulation and conception, one should follow a balanced diet that promotes insulin sensitivity, hormone balance, and a healthy weight.

Managing PCOS symptoms and enhancing general health and wellbeing can be accomplished by implementing a nutrient-dense diet that emphasizes whole, unprocessed foods, an abundance of fruits and vegetables, lean proteins, healthy fats, and complex carbohydrates

Chapter two

List of foods that are good for PCOS

A summary of foods that are good for PCOS includes a range of nutrient-dense choices that can assist with managing symptoms and promoting general health and wellbeing. These are the main food classes that are beneficial for PCOS:

1.lean Proteins:
- Poultry (turkey, chicken)
- Fish (tuna, trout, and salmon)
- Trimmed meat or pork portions
- Eggs
- Legumes (beans, lentils, and

chickpeas), tofu, and tempeh are examples of plant-based proteins.

2.High-Fibre Foods:

• Whole grains, such as oats, barley, quinoa, and brown rice

• Fruits, particularly pears, apples, and berries

• Vegetables, such as cauliflower, broccoli, Brussels sprouts, and leafy greens

• Nuts and seeds, such as flaxseeds, chia seeds, and almonds

3.Healthy Fats:

• Lawyers

• Seeds and nuts

• Olive oil

• Oily fish, such as sardines, mackerel, and salmon

- Moderate use of coconut oil

4.Carbohydrates with a low Glycemic:

- Sugar potatoes
- A whole grains, for example quinoa, brown rice, and whole wheat
- Legumes (lentils, beans)
- Non-starchy veggies, such as bell peppers, broccoli, and leafy greens

5.Anti-Inflammation food:

- Omega-3 fatty acid-rich fatty fish
- Berries, such as raspberries, strawberries, and blueberries
- Leafy greens (kale, spinach)
- Ginger
- Ginger

6.Dairy substitutes (for people who are sensitive to dairy or have lactose intolerance):

• Soy, coconut milk, or un-sweetened almond milk

• Yogurt without dairy made with soy, coconut, or almond milk

7.Particular Supplements for PCOS:

• Inositol: A substance that resembles a B vitamin and may help control menstrual cycles and insulin sensitivity.

• Vitamin D: Beneficial for general health and may lessen PCOS symptoms.

• Omega-3 fatty acids: These anti-inflammatory fats, which can be found in fatty fish and supplements, may help control the symptoms of PCOS.

8. Hydration

• Water is necessary for hydration and general wellness. Throughout the day, it's critical to maintain a sufficient water intake in order to manage PCOS symptoms.

9. Limiting Sugar-Sweet and Processed Foods:

• Reduce your consumption of processed foods, candies, pastries, and sugar-filled beverages because these can raise blood sugar levels and cause insulin resistance.

People with PCOS can manage their weight, enhance insulin sensitivity, lower inflammation, and support hormone balance by including these PCOS-friendly foods in a balanced diet. These benefits are crucial for controlling PCOS symptoms and enhancing general health.

Chapter three

List of foods that people with PCOS should limit or stay away from

Certain foods may make symptoms of PCOS (polycystic ovary syndrome) worse or worsen underlying metabolic imbalances in those who have it. The following foods should be limited or avoided:

1.Sugar-filled Foods and Drinks:

• Cola

• Fruit juices enhanced with sugar

• Sweetened coffee and tea beverages

• Chocolates, candies, and

confections

• Refined sugar-containing
pastries, cakes, cookies, and
other baked foods

2.Highly Processed Foods:

• Quick food

• Snacks in a package, such as
cookies, crackers, and chips

• Processed meats like sausages
and hot dogs, as well as frozen
dinners

• Pre-packaged meals and instant
noodles that are heavy in sodium
and preservatives

**3.Carbohydrates with a high
Glycemic index:**

• White bread

• White rice

• Sugar-filled cereals

- Instant oatmeal with sweeteners added
- Standard spaghetti

4.Trans fats and saturated fats:

- Fried food items
- Meat cuts high in fat
- Dairy products with added fat, such as butter and cheese
- Other hydrogenated oils and margarine
- Processed beef, for instance sausage and bacon

5.Overindulgence in Coffee:

- Although some PCOS sufferers may tolerate a moderate amount of coffee, excessive caffeine consumption might upset the hormone balance and worsen symptoms like anxiety and insomnia.

6.Alcohol

• Drinking too much alcohol can have a detrimental effect on hormone metabolism and liver function, aggravating PCOS symptoms. Take little alcohol or abstain from it completely.

7. Dairy Products: (for certain people)

• Lactose intolerance or sensitivity to dairy products may be present in certain PCOS-affected women, which might worsen gastrointestinal symptoms or increase inflammation. If dairy bothers you, try soy milk, coconut milk, or almond milk as dairy substitutes.

8.Foods High in Sodium:

• Processed foods such as sauces, condiments, and soups in cans

• Carved and prepared meats

• Salty appetizers such as pretzels and chips

• Sodium-laden fast food and restaurant meals

Chapter four

Choosing a healthy breakfast menu

Here are some healthy breakfast ideas that are appropriate for people with PCOS:

1.Greek Yogurt Concession:

• Greek yogurt without added sugar

• Recently harvested berries, like raspberries, blueberries, and strawberries

• Ground flaxseeds or chia seeds

• An optional honey drizzle or cinnamon sprinkle

• Almonds or granola for crunch (if desired)

2.Vegetable Omelette:

• Eggs (egg whites or whole)

• Diced veggies, such as onions, mushrooms, bell peppers, and spinach

• Goat or Feta cheese (optional)

• Fresh herbs, such basil or parsley

• Avocado slices or whole grain bread on the side

3.Oats for Overnight:

• Old-fashioned oats, or rolled oats

• Almond or coconut milk without sugar

• Ground flaxseeds or chia seeds

• Cut berries or bananas

• Nut butter, cinnamon, and vanilla extract are optional add-ins.

• Store in the refrigerator
overnight and eat cold or warm
the next day.

4. Smoothie Bowl:

• Mixed frozen berries,
comprising raspberries,
blueberries, and strawberries.

• Leaves of kale or spinach

• Almond milk or coconut water
without added sugar

• For extra protein, try Greek
yogurt or protein powder.

• Garnish with chopped banana,
granola, shredded coconut,
almonds, and seeds.

5. Toast with avocados:

• Whole grain toast (bread)

• Avocado mashed and seasoned

with salt, pepper, and lemon juice

• Cut up radishes or tomatoes

• An optional sprinkle of
nutritional yeast or feta cheese

• Top with scrambled or poached
eggs for extra protein.

6.Breakfast Bowl with Quinoa:

• Prepared quinoa

• Cherry tomatoes with sautéed
greens, such as spinach and kale

• Fried or poached egg on top

• Feta cheese or nutritional yeast
sprinkled on top

• A small drop of balsamic
vinegar and olive oil

7.Pudding with Chia Seeds:

• Chia seeds

• Almond or coconut milk without
sugar

- For sweetness, a little honey or maple syrup combined with vanilla extract
- Ripe berries or pieces of fresh fruit to garnish
- Chopped almonds or coconut flakes are optional.

These healthy, well-balanced breakfast options can help people with PCOS manage their blood sugar, control their hunger, and maintain their general health.

Sample recipes include egg-based meals, overnight oats, and smoothie bowls.

Of course! Here are some example meals that highlight

nutrition and balance for those with PCOS and include smoothie bowls, overnight oats, and egg-based dishes:

1.Bowl of Smoothies: Berry Blast

Components:

• One cup of mixed berries, comprising raspberries, blueberries, and strawberries

• One ripe banana

• Half a cup of spinach leaves

• 1/2 cup of plain Greek yogurt

• 1 tablespoon chia seed

• 1/4 cup unsweetened almond milk

Toppings

• A banana, sliced

• Granola

- Coconut shreds

- Diced seeds or nuts

Guidelines:

1. Blend together mixed berries, almond milk, banana, spinach, Greek yogurt, and chia seeds in a blender.

2. Blend until creamy and smooth.

3. Transfer the blended drink to a bowl.

4. Add chopped nuts or seeds, granola, shredded coconut, and banana slices on top.

5. Eat it right away with a spoon!

2.Nighttime Oats: Nut-Crusted Banana Delight

ingredient:

- 1/2 a cup of rolled or old-fashioned oats

• 1/2 cup almond milk without sugar

• Mashed 1 ripe banana

• 1 tablespoon chia seed

• 1/4 teaspoon vanilla extract

• Dash of cinnamon (optional)

Toppings:

• A banana, sliced

• Chopped nuts (almonds, walnuts, or pecans)

• sprinkle of honey or maple syrup (but optional)

Guidelines:

1. In a jar or container, combine rolled oats, almond milk, mashed banana, chia seeds, vanilla extract, and cinnamon (if using).

2. Stir well to combine all

ingredients.

3. Cover and refrigerate overnight, or for at least 4 hours, to allow the oats to soften and absorb the liquid.

4. In the morning, give the oats a stir and add additional almond milk if desired for desired consistency.

5. Top with sliced banana, chopped nuts, and a drizzle of honey or maple syrup if desired.

6. Enjoy cold straight from the fridge!

3. Egg-Based Dish: Veggie Frittata

Ingredient:

- 6 eggs
- 1/4 cup milk (or unsweetened

almond milk)

- 1 cup mixed vegetables (spinach, bell peppers, onions, mushrooms)
- 1/2 cup cherry tomatoes, halved
- 1/4 cup crumbled feta cheese (optional)
- Salt and pepper to taste
- Olive oil for cooking

Guidelines:

1.Preheat the oven to 350°F (175°C).

2.put in a bowl, whisk together eggs, milk, salt, and pepper until well together.

3. Heat olive oil in an oven-safe skillet over medium heat.

4. Add mixed vegetables and

sauté until softened, about 5 minutes.

5. Pour the egg mixture over the vegetables in the skillet.

6. Scatter cherry tomatoes and crumbled feta cheese (if using) over the top.

7. Cook on the stovetop for 3-4 minutes until the edges begin to set.

8. Transfer the skillet to the preheated oven and bake for 15-20 minutes, or until the frittata is set in the center and lightly golden on top.

9. Bring out from the oven and let it cool slightly before slicing.

10. Serve warm or at room temperature, and enjoy a slice of

veggie frittata for breakfast!

These recipes offer a variety of flavors and textures while providing balanced nutrition to support individuals with PCOS in managing their symptoms and promoting overall health and well-being. Adjust ingredients and toppings according to personal preferences and dietary needs.

Chapter five

Variety of satisfying meals for lunch and dinner

Of course! Here are some satisfying lunch and dinner meal ideas for individuals with PCOS, incorporating a balance of protein, healthy fats, and complex carbohydrates:

1.Grilled Salmon with Quinoa Salad:

• Grilled salmon fillets seasoned with lemon, garlic, and herbs.

• Quinoa salad with diced cucumbers, cherry tomatoes, red onions, and chopped fresh herbs (such as parsley or mint). Garnish

with, lemon juice, salt, pepper
and olive oil.

• Steamed or roasted vegetables,
such as broccoli, cauliflower, or
asparagus, seasoned with olive
oil, garlic, and herbs.

2. Turkey and Avocado Wrap:

• Whole grain or spinach wrap
filled with sliced turkey breast,
mashed avocado, lettuce, tomato,
and cucumber.

• Side of raw veggie sticks
(carrots, bell peppers, celery)
with hummus for dipping.

• Mixed green salad with a
vinaigrette dressing made from
olive oil, balsamic vinegar, Dijon
mustard, and herbs.

3. Vegetable Stir-Fry with

Tofu:

• Stir-fried tofu cubes with mixed vegetables (bell peppers, broccoli, snap peas, carrots, and mushrooms) in a ginger-garlic sauce.

• serve with brown rice or cauliflower rice for a low carb choice.

• Garnish your veg with chopped green onions and sesame seeds.

4. Mediterranean Salad with Chickpeas:

• Diced cucumbers, cherry tomatoes, red onions, crumbled feta cheese, and Kalamata olives combined with the chickpeas.

• A dressing consisting of garlic, oregano, olive oil, lemon juice, salt, and pepper.

• You may serve it with whole grain pita bread or on a bed of mixed greens.

5. Grilled chicken and pesto-sauced zucchini noodles:

• Homemade basil pesto (prepared with basil, pine nuts, garlic, Parmesan cheese, olive oil, salt, and pepper) served with zucchini noodles, or zoodles.

• Slices of grill-seasoned chicken breast seasoned with Italian herbs.

• Roasted cherry tomato side with cloves of garlic.

6. Tacos with black beans and vegetables:

• Black beans, diced tomatoes, onions, and bell peppers sautéed in whole grain or corn tortillas.

• Garnished with slices of avocado, salsa, and a dollop of sour cream or Greek yogurt.

• Garnish with lime juice and serve alongside brown rice.

7. Stuffed bell peppers with ground turkey and quinoa:

• Halved bell peppers filled with a blend of chopped tomatoes, black beans, corn, cooked quinoa, and lean ground turkey seasoning.

• Bake until the filling is thoroughly cooked and the peppers are soft.

• Add some chopped cilantro and Greek yogurt as garnishes.

These meal plans include balanced nutrition and a range of flavors and textures to help people with PCOS manage their symptoms and enhance their general health and well-being. Take into account dietary requirements and personal tastes while adjusting ingredients and seasonings.

Including nutritious grains, lean proteins, and a plenty of vegetables

Of course! Let's develop PCOS-friendly lunch and dinner alternatives that include lean proteins, nutritious grains, and an abundance of vegetables:

1. Lunch would be grilled chicken with quinoa salad.

• Lean Protein: Marinated chicken breast on the grill with herbs, olive oil, and lemon juice.

• Whole Grains: A quinoa salad flavored with sliced bell peppers, cucumbers, and cherry tomatoes, along with fresh herbs like basil or parsley.

• An plenty of veggies: Top the quinoa salad with spinach or mixed greens and serve it with roasted or steamed vegetables on the side.

2. Dinner is roasted vegetables and brown rice with baked salmon.

• Lean Protein: Dill, garlic, and lemon-seasoned baked salmon fillets.

• Whole Grains: To enhance flavor, boil brown rice in water or vegetable broth.

• An abundance of veggies, including roasted mixed vegetables with garlic, olive oil, and herbs, such as Brussels sprouts, cauliflower, broccoli, and carrots.

3. Lunch is a whole grain wrap with turkey and avocado.

• Lean Protein: A wrap made of healthy grains or spinach with sliced turkey breast within.

• Whole Grains: For the basis, use whole grain sandwich bread or wrap.

• Ample Vegetables: Stuff the wrap with sliced cucumber, tomato, lettuce, avocado, and any other preferred vegetables. Accompany with a mixed greens side salad.

4. Supper is quinoa and a veggie stir-fry with tofu.

Lean protein can be found in stir-fried tofu cubes with carrots, broccoli, snap peas, and bell peppers in a soy-ginger sauce.

• Whole Grains: To add more protein and fiber to cooked quinoa, serve the veggie stir-fry on top of it.

• An abundance of Vegetables: For extra nutrition, add a ton of vibrant vegetables to the stir-fry.

5. Lunch is grilled shrimp served with a spinach and chickpea salad.

• Lean Protein: Garlic, paprika, and lemon seasoning grilled shrimp.

• Whole Grains: Toss cooked farro or quinoa with chopped feta cheese, cherry tomatoes, red onions, and chickpeas in a spinach salad.

• An abundance of vegetables: Avocado, bell peppers, cucumbers, and spinach all contribute flavor and texture to a dish while providing a nutrient-rich base.

6. Dinner is a brown basmati rice curry with lentils and vegetables.

• Lean Protein: To make a tasty vegetarian protein source, sauté lentils with onions, garlic, ginger, and curry spices.

• Whole Grains: For a filling and wholesome supper, serve the lentil curry over cooked brown basmati rice.

• An abundance of veggies: To add texture and nutrients, include a variety of vegetables in the curry, such as bell peppers, carrots, cauliflower, and spinach.

Chapter six

Recipe samples for salads, grain bowls, stir-fries, and soups

1. Salad made with Mediterranean chickpeas

Ingredient:

• One can of washed and drained chickpeas

• One diced cucumber

• Half a cup of cherry tomatoes

• 1/4 cup coarsely chopped red onion

• 1/4 cup sliced Kalamata olives

• Two tablespoons of feta cheese, crumbled

• Two tablespoons of freshly chopped parsley

• To dress, combine 2 tablespoons extra virgin olive oil, 1 tablespoon lemon juice, 1 teaspoon Dijon mustard and salt and pepper to taste.

Guidelines:

1. Chickpeas, cucumber, cherry tomatoes, red onion, olives, and parsley should all be combined in a big bowl.

2.To create the dressing, combine the olive oil, lemon juice, Dijon mustard, salt, and pepper in a small bowl.

3. Drizzle the salad with the dressing and toss to coat.

4. Before serving, scatter the feta cheese on top.

2. Stir-Fry: Stir-fried Tofu with Veggies

ingredient:

• One block of pressed and cubed extra-firm tofu

• Two cups of mixed veggies, such as carrots, snap peas, broccoli, and bell peppers

• Two minced garlic cloves

• Twice as much soy sauce

• Tsp of sesame oil

• One tablespoon of cornstarch, if desired, to thicken the sauce

• Prepared quinoa or brown rice for serving

Guidelines:

1. In a large skillet or wok, heat the sesame oil over medium-high heat.

2. Tofu cubes should be added and cooked until golden brown all over. place aside from the skillet when taken out.

3. Add minced garlic and mixed vegetables to the same skillet. fry the vegetable till they become crisp-tender.

4. Combine the soy sauce and cornstarch (if desired) in a small bowl. After adding the sauce, simmer the vegetables until it thickens.

5. Return the cooked tofu to the skillet and mix everything together.

6. Serve the cooked quinoa or brown rice with the tofu and veggie stir-fry.

3. Soup: Vegetable and Lentil Soup

ingredient:

• One cup of rinsed dried green or brown lentils

• One chopped onion

- Two diced carrots

- Two chopped celery stalks

- Two minced garlic cloves

- Diced tomatoes, one can

- Four cups broth made of
vegetables

- One tsp. dried thyme

- Add pepper and salt to taste.

- If desired, fresh parsley for
garnish

Guidelines:

1. Warm up the olive oil in a big
pot over medium heat. Add the
minced garlic, celery, carrots, and
onion. stir fry the veggies till they
get tender.

2. To the pot, add diced tomatoes, vegetable broth, dry thyme, and lentils. Add pepper and salt for seasoning.

3. Once the soup is boiling, lower the heat and simmer it for twenty to twenty-five minutes, or until the lentils are soft.

4. If necessary, taste and adjust the seasoning.

4. Quinoa and Roasted Vegetable Bowl - Grain Bowl

Ingredient:

- A cup of quinoa, cooked

- One cup of mixed roasted vegetables, such as cauliflower,

Brussels sprouts, and sweet
potatoes

• Half a cup of cooked lentils

• Two cups of mixed greens
(kale, spinach, and arugula)

• 1/4 cup of feta cheese,
crumbled

• To dress, combine 2
tablespoons extra virgin olive oil,
1 tablespoon balsamic vinegar, 1
teaspoon honey, and your desired
amount of salt and pepper.

Guidelines:

1. Put cooked quinoa, cooked
chickpeas, roasted veggies, and
mixed greens in a big bowl.

2. To make the dressing, combine the olive oil, balsamic vinegar, honey, salt, and pepper in a small bowl.

3. Toss to coat the quinoa and vegetable mixture after adding the dressing.

4. Before serving, scatter some crumbled feta cheese over the top.

Lean proteins, whole grains, and an abundance of veggies are combined in these sample recipes to provide a delicious and healthy range of salad, stir-fry, soup, and grain bowl alternatives that will help people with PCOS manage their symptoms and enhance their general health and well-being. Take into account dietary requirements and personal tastes while adjusting ingredients and seasonings.

Suggestions for nutritious snacks to quell cravings

Here are some suggestions for nutritious foods that will satisfy cravings and help PCOS sufferers control their symptoms:

1. Greek Yogurt with Berries: Greek yogurt is a filling snack option because it is low in sugar and high in protein. For extra fiber and antioxidants, sprinkle some fresh berries, such as raspberries, blueberries, or strawberries, on top.

2. Crunchy veggies like carrots, cucumbers, bell peppers, and celery may be sliced up and dipped in hummus to make a filling snack that's high in vitamins, minerals, and fiber.

3. Hard-Boiled Eggs: Packed with protein, vitamins, and minerals, hard-boiled eggs are a handy and transportable snack choice. For added taste, season them with a little salt and pepper.

4. Mixed Nuts: A tiny handful of mixed nuts, such pistachios, almonds, and walnuts, can supply fiber, protein, and healthy fats to

keep you feeling full in between
meals. Just watch how much you
eat to limit your calorie intake.

5. Edamame: Packed full of
protein, fiber, and antioxidants,
steamed edamame (young
soybeans) is a healthy snack
choice. For extra taste, add a
little chile flakes or sea salt.

6. Cottage Cheese with Fruit:
Protein and calcium are abundant
in cottage cheese. Serve it with
sliced melon, pineapple, or
peaches for a tasty and sweet
snack.

7. Avocado Toast: For a tasty
and filling snack high in fiber and
healthy fats, spread mashed

avocado on whole grain toast and top with sliced tomatoes, feta cheese, and a drizzle of balsamic sauce.

8. Roasted Chickpeas: For a crunchy and tasty snack that is high in protein and fiber, roast chickpeas in the oven with a little olive oil and your favorite spices (such as paprika, cumin, or garlic powder) until crispy.

9. Dark Chocolate Covered Almonds: Treat your sweet craving to a tiny portion of almonds covered in dark chocolate. Almonds offer protein and good lipids, while dark chocolate is a great source of antioxidants.

10. Apple Slices with Nut Butter: For a filling and healthy snack that blends sweetness with protein and good fats, slice up an apple and spread each slice with your favorite nut butter (such peanut butter or almond butter).

Techniques for creating enticing desserts with PCOS-friendly components

Of course! Choosing options that are high in fiber, low in added sugars, and contain components that promote hormone balance and blood sugar regulation are all important when creating satiating sweet treats with PCOS-friendly ingredients. Here are a few tactics and concepts:

1. Natural Sweeteners: Sweeten your delights with natural sweeteners sparingly rather than refined sugars, such as honey, maple syrup, or stevia. These choices can lessen blood sugar rises since they have a lower glycemic index.

2. Whole Grain Flours: Rather than using refined white flour, use whole grain flours like oat flour, coconut flour, or almond flour. Because these substitutes have more protein and fiber, their blood sugar levels may be more stabilized.

3. Nuts, seeds, and avocados are good sources of fat, so include them in your baked goods. Good fats have the ability to lower blood sugar and promote satiety.

4. Fiber-Rich components: To help slow down the absorption of sugar into the bloodstream and encourage feelings of fullness, use fiber-rich components like fruits, vegetables, and legumes in your sweet treats. Berries, apples, pumpkin, and black beans are a few examples.

5. Protein Boost: Include protein in your sweets to improve satiety and blood sugar regulation. Excellent options for including protein in dishes are Greek yogurt, cottage cheese, protein powder, and nuts or seeds.

6. Portion Control: To prevent consuming too many calories and sugar, watch how much you eat when you like sweets. Pay attention to your body's signals of hunger and fullness as you carefully savor your goodies.

7. Balanced dishes: To assist maintain stable blood sugar levels and encourage overall satisfaction, look for dishes that offer a balance of healthy fats, proteins, and carbohydrates.

Keeping these tactics in mind, here are some scrumptious dessert recipes made using PCOS-friendly ingredients:

- **Berry Chia Seed Pudding:** Blend unsweetened almond milk, fresh berries, a small amount of honey or maple syrup, and chia seeds. To make it thicker, refrigerate it for an entire night. Garnish with more berries and a scattering of nuts or seeds before serving.

- **Banana Oat Cookies:** Mash ripe bananas and combine with rolled oats, chopped almonds or dark chocolate chips, and a pinch of cinnamon. Transfer onto an oven tray and cook for a golden hue.

- **Greek Yogurt Parfait:** To add crunch, layer Greek yogurt with sliced fruits, such as mangoes, peaches, or berries, then top with chopped almonds or granola.

- **Make your own Energy Bites** by combining nut butter, honey, maple syrup, rolled oats, and dried fruit, chia seeds, and shredded coconut as mix-ins. Form into little balls and place in the refrigerator to solidify.

- **Avocado Chocolate Mousse:** Until smooth and creamy, blend ripe avocado, cocoa powder, a small amount of honey or maple syrup, and a splash of almond milk. Present cold, accompanied by a dollop of Greek yogurt or fluffy coconut cream.

In order to promote general health and wellbeing, these ideas for sweet treats include tasty selections that are higher in fiber, lower in added sugars, and contain PCOS-friendly components. You are welcome to alter recipes to fit your dietary requirements and taste preferences.

Chapter seven

Examples of recipes include fruit-based sweets, veggie sticks with dip, and energy nibbles.

Of course! Here are some example recipes employing PCOS-friendly ingredients for fruit-based desserts, veggie sticks with dip, and energy bites:

1. Energy Bits:

Ingredient:

• One cup of rolled oats

• Half a cup of natural nut butter, like peanut or almond butter

• 1/4 cup maple syrup or honey

• Two tsp of chia seed

- 1/4 cup chocolate chips, dark

- ¼ cup chopped nuts walnuts or almonds

- One tsp vanilla extract

- A dash of salt

Guidelines:

1. Rolling oats, nut butter, honey or maple syrup, chia seeds, chocolate chips, chopped nuts, vanilla essence, and a dash of salt should all be combined in a mixing basin.

2. Stir the mixture until it comes together and is well blended.

3. using your hands, roll the mixture into bite-sized balls.

4. To make the energy bites firmer, place them on a baking sheet covered with parchment paper and chill for at least half an hour.

5. When the energy bites are solid, move them to an airtight container and keep them in the fridge for up to a week.

6. Savor as a wholesome on-the-go snack!

2. Carrot sticks dipped in dip:

Ingredient:

- A variety of veggies, including celery, bell peppers, cucumbers, and carrots

- Regarding the dip:

• 1/2 cup of plain Greek yogurt

• Two tahini tablespoons.

• A tsp of lemon juice

• Finely chopped garlic clove

• Add pepper and salt to taste.

• Chopped fresh herbs (such dill or parsley) are optional.

Guidelines:

1. Slices or sticks of various veggies should be chopped after washing.

2. Greek yogurt, tahini, lemon juice, minced garlic, salt, and pepper should all be combined smoothly in a small bowl.

3. If desired, add finely chopped fresh herbs.

4. Serve the dip alongside the vegetable sticks for a crisp and filling snack.

3. Fruit-Based Dessert:

Coconut Chia Berry Pudding:

ingredient:

4.25 cups of chia seeds

• One cup of almond milk without sugar

• 1 tablespoon of maple honey or syrup

• Half a teaspoon of essence from vanilla

• Half a cup of mixed berries, including raspberries, blueberries, and strawberries

• Two tablespoons of coconut shreds

Guidelines:

1. Chia seeds, unsweetened almond milk, vanilla extract, and honey or maple syrup should all be combined in a bowl. Mix thoroughly to blend.

2. To avoid clumping, whisk the mixture once more after letting it sit for about ten minutes.

3. To enable the chia seeds to soak up the liquid and thicken, cover the bowl and place it in the

refrigerator for at least two hours or overnight.

4. After the chia pudding sets, fill serving glasses or bowls with layers of mixed berries and shredded coconut.

5. Serve cold as a tasty and wholesome fruit-based snack or dessert.

With PCOS-friendly ingredients, these sample recipes provide tasty and fulfilling options for fruit-based desserts, veggie sticks with dip, and energy nibbles. You are welcome to alter the recipes to fit your dietary requirements and taste preferences by adding your own flavors and ingredients.

As part of a balanced diet that promotes general health and wellbeing, savor these nourishing snacks.

Talk about PCOS-friendly and hydrating drink alternatives

Everyone, even those with PCOS, needs to drink enough water. Maintaining adequate hydration facilitates digestion, controls body temperature, and supports good skin. It's critical to choose drinks that not only hydrate but also help manage PCOS by staying away from excessively caffeinated and added sugars. The following is a list of hydrating and PCOS-friendly drinks:

1. Water: With no calories, sugar, or additives, water is the ideal option for staying hydrated. It's important to maintain proper biological functions and hydration levels by consuming enough water throughout the day. Try to consume eight glasses (64 ounces) of water or more if you live in a hot area or are physically active each day.

2. Herbal Teas: A calming substitute for caffeinated beverages, herbal teas are hydrating. Select herbal teas that are naturally caffeine-free, such as those made from peppermint, chamomile, ginger, or rooibos.

Herbal teas can support antioxidants, aid in digestion, and encourage relaxation.

3. Infused Water: Adding natural flavor to water by infusing it with fresh fruits, vegetables, or herbs doesn't include extra calories or sugar. For a cool and hydrating drink alternative, try infusing water with pieces of citrus fruits (such lemon, lime, or orange), cucumber, berries, mint, or basil.

4. Coconut Water: Rich in electrolytes like potassium, magnesium, and calcium, coconut water is a naturally occurring hydrating choice that is particularly beneficial after physical activity or in hot weather. For the healthiest option, go for basic coconut water that hasn't had any tastes or sugar added.

5. Sparkling Water: A delightful substitute for sugar-filled sodas and carbonated drinks, sparkling water offers hydration with a frothy texture. Choose sparkling water that doesn't have any artificial sweeteners or added sugars, and drink it either simple or with a squeeze of citrus.

6. Green Tea: Rich in antioxidants, green tea is a PCOS-friendly beverage option that may help reduce inflammation and insulin resistance. Green tea is a more hydrating beverage when either hot or cold, and it has less caffeine than coffee.

7. Homemade Smoothies: A healthy and hydrating beverage option can be a homemade smoothie made with unsweetened almond milk, water, or coconut water mixed with fruits, vegetables, and protein sources like Greek yogurt or protein powder. Steer clear of adding too many sugars or sugary foods.

8. Drinking fermented tea in moderation can help promote gut health as it includes probiotics. Kombucha is a type of tea. To reduce added sugars, go for unsweetened or mildly sweetened types. Consume kombucha in moderation as part of a healthy diet.

Ideas for smoothies, infused water, and herbal teas

1. Herbal Teas:

• Peppermint Tea: This refreshing tea is a fantastic alternative after meals since it can help calm digestion.

• Chamomile Tea: Due to its relaxing qualities, chamomile tea may aid in improving sleep quality and relaxation.

• Ginger Tea: This hot beverage helps soothe inflammation and improve digestion. It's excellent for relieving upset stomachs as well.

• Rooibos Tea: This tasty and hydrating tea is devoid of caffeine and high in antioxidants.

• Hibiscus Tea: Rich in antioxidants, hibiscus tea is tart and refreshing and may help decrease blood pressure and promote heart health.

2. Water With Infusion:

• Citrus Mint Infused Water: For a zesty and cooling infusion, combine orange, lemon, and lime segments with fresh mint leaves.

• Cucumber Basil Infused Water: To add a refreshing and herbaceous flavor to water, add cucumber slices and fresh basil leaves.

• Berry Blast Infused Water: For a delightful and vibrant infusion, combine water with strawberries, blueberries, and raspberries.

• Watermelon Mint Infused Water: For a refreshing and summertime beverage, blend watermelon chunks with fresh mint leaves. Then, combine the mixture with water.

• Pineapple Coconut Infused Water: For a refreshing and tropical infusion, blend chunks of pineapple with coconut water.

3. Smoothies:

• Green Goddess Smoothie: For a nutrient-rich and hydrating green smoothie, blend spinach, kale, cucumber, green apple, Greek yogurt, and a small amount of coconut water.

• Berry Blast Smoothie: This tasty and antioxidant-rich smoothie is made with mixed berries (strawberries, blueberries, and raspberries), banana, spinach, almond milk, and a scoop of protein powder.

• Tropical Paradise Smoothie: For a cool, tropical-flavored smoothie, blend mango, pineapple, banana, coconut water, and a small handful of spinach.

• Rich and filling smoothie full of fiber and healthy fats: Blend avocado, banana, spinach, almond milk, and a scoop of vanilla protein powder.

• Chocolate Peanut Butter Smoothie: For a rich and high-protein smoothie, blend unsweetened cocoa powder, banana, peanut butter, spinach, almond milk, and a scoop of protein powder.

These recipes for smoothies, infused water, and herbal teas provide a range of tasty and hydrating choices that include PCOS-friendly ingredients. You are welcome to alter the recipes to suit your dietary requirements and taste preferences. Savor these drinks as a component of a well-rounded diet to promote general health and wellbeing as well as hydration.

Chapter eight

Advice for cutting back on alcohol and sugary drinks

Reducing alcohol and sugary drink intake is crucial for overall health, especially for PCOS patients who may be more susceptible to blood sugar swings and hormone abnormalities. The following advice may be used to lower intake:

1. Be Aware of Portion Sizes: Take caution when consuming alcohol or sugar-filled beverages. To cut down on your overall consumption of alcohol and added sugars, stick to smaller servings.

2. Read Labels: Look for information on added sugars and alcohol amounts on beverage labels. When selecting a beverage, try to find options with less sugar or without artificial sweeteners.

3. Make Water Your Main Drink of Choice: Throughout the day, make water your go-to beverage. Reusable water bottles can help you keep hydrated and resist the need to go for sugary or alcoholic beverages.

4. Limit Sugary Drinks: Cut back on the amount of sugary beverages you consume, including fruit juices, sodas, energy drinks, and teas with added sugar. Instead, go for infused water, herbal drinks, or plain water.

5. Make Your Own Drinks: Using natural ingredients, make at-home substitutes for alcoholic and sugary drinks. Try out different flavor combos and recipes to make hydrating and refreshing drinks at home.

6. Sugary Drinks: If you want your drinks sweetened, you can cut the sugar amount without sacrificing flavor by diluting them with water or sparkling water.

7. Limit Alcohol Intake: When drinking, consider reduced alcohol options and keep your intake to a minimum. Pay attention to portion sizes and refrain from overindulging, since this may have detrimental impacts on hormone balance, blood sugar regulation, and general health.

8. Set Personal Limits and Objectives: Decide on your own personal alcohol and sugary drink intake limits and objectives. Establish a weekly intake limit that you are comfortable with and adhere to it.

9. Practice proportion: As part of a balanced diet, indulge in alcohol and sugary drinks in proportion. Consuming nutrient-dense foods and drinks that promote general health and wellbeing should be your main priority.

10. Seek Support: Consult with friends, family, or a healthcare provider for assistance if you're having trouble cutting back on alcohol or sugar-filled beverages. They can offer you support, responsibility, and direction to help you reach your objectives.

You may support your health and well-being by reducing your consumption of alcohol and sugary drinks and by giving priority to hydrating and PCOS-friendly beverage options. Always

keep in mind to find the tactics
that are most effective for you
and your lifestyle, and to make
adjustments gradually.

Advice on meal preparation and planning for PCOS sufferers

For those with PCOS, meal
planning and preparation can help
maintain balanced nutrition,
control blood sugar, and advance
general health and wellbeing.
Here are some tips for food
preparation and planning
specifically for those with PCOS:

**1. Emphasis on Balanced
Meals:** To assist stabilize blood
sugar levels and encourage

fullness, try to include a balance of healthy fats, proteins, and carbohydrates in each meal. Whenever possible, opt for whole, minimally processed foods.

2. Lean Protein Sources: Include sources of lean protein in your meals, such as fish, chicken, tofu, tempeh, lentils, and low-fat dairy products. Foods high in protein can improve muscular function, control blood sugar levels, and control hunger.

3. Select Complex carbs: To assist sustain consistent energy levels and encourage feelings of fullness, choose complex carbs that are high in fiber and low in added sugars. Whole grains like quinoa, brown rice, oats, and whole wheat pasta are a few examples, along with starchy veggies like peas, sweet potatoes, and squash.

4. Make Healthy Fats Your Top Priority: Include foods high in healthy fats in your meals, such as avocados, almonds, seeds, olive oil, and fatty fish (sardines, mackerel, and salmon). The synthesis of hormones, the health of the brain, and the absorption of nutrients all depend on healthy fats.

5. Stress Plant-Based Foods: To boost fiber consumption, supply vital vitamins and minerals, and promote general health, include a lot of fruits, vegetables, and plant-based foods in your meals. Try to assemble colorful fruits and vegetables to cover half of your platter.

6. Eat Less Processed meals and Added Sugars: Reduce the amount of meals and drinks that are heavy in processed components, added sugars, and refined carbohydrates. These may worsen the symptoms of PCOS by causing insulin resistance, inflammation, and blood sugar increases.

7. Plan Ahead: Give your weekly meal and snack schedule some thought. Make sure you have all the products you need on hand by making a grocery list based on your meal plan. Making a plan ahead of time can support healthy eating habits, save time, and lower stress.

8. preparing in Bulk: If you want to have plenty of grains, meats, and veggies for the week, think about preparing them in big quantities. Meal preparation can be streamlined by prepping items ahead of time, which also makes it simpler to put together wholesome meals quickly on hectic days.

9. Experiment with Recipes: To keep meals engaging and pleasurable, try out new recipes and play around with flavors, cuisines, and cooking methods. Seek for meals that are good for PCOS and highlight nutrient-dense foods and natural foods.

10. Listen to Your Body: Take note of the effects that various foods have on your body and modify your meal plan as necessary. Make an effort to fuel your body with foods that give you a sense of balance, satiety, and energy.